Diabetic Diet: 30-Day Lifestyle Plan To Maintain A Healthy Weight

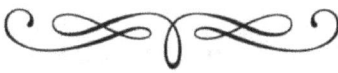

Weight Loss and Healthy Diet Plan For Diabetics

By

Jamie Tyler

TABLE OF CONTENT

Introduction

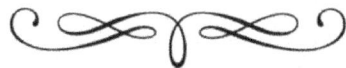

This book contains proven steps and strategies on how to help you curb and control one of the major lifestyle diseases, **Diabetes**.

Today, more and more people are getting affected by diabetes. It is like there is an epidemic of diabetes! **But, did you know that most of the cases of diabetes could have been prevented, if the affected would have tweaked their lifestyle a little bit?**

Most people get this mental image of starving and giving up their favorite foods in order to prevent and control diabetes. Yes, consuming the right foods is important, but you really don't need to give up your all favorite desserts or resort to eating bland food to be healthy.

Even if you don't have diabetes, it is extremely important for you follow a healthy life style, eat the correct food and do the correct activities, so that you do not get the disease.

Well, if you do have diabetes, relax. It is not the end of the world! Regularly check your diabetes, eat right and exercise well, making the correct life style choices may even reverse your diabetes!

In this book I will talk about what diabetes is, the effect the disease has on your body, the different types of diabetes, the foods you (as a diabetic) should consume, the foods you should avoid, physical activities you should undertake and of course a 30-day suggested meal plan **(but before you embark on any diet plan please consult your physician).**

I thank you for downloading this book and sincerely wish that the information provided in this book helps you make life changing choices and opens the doors for a healthier tomorrow.

Jamie Tyler

Chapter 1: What Is Diabetes?

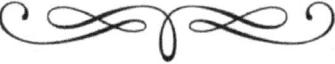

Diabetes!! The word is enough to send shivers down anyone's spine, especially a dessert lover's! But do we actually know what diabetes is?

Diabetes mellitus, commonly just known as diabetes, is not just one disease. No, it is a group of metabolic diseases. The most common and widely known effect of this disease is elevated blood sugar levels for an extended period of time.

But what exactly happens in diabetes?

Diabetes is a disorder of the metabolism. Metabolism is the way our body breaks down our food and uses it for growth and energy purposes. A lot of what we eat is digested to glucose, which is the most essential source of energy for our body.

Glucose from the digested food is pushed into our bloodstream and is used to provide energy for our day-to-day activities. But, the glucose cannot enter our bloodstream without insulin. **Insulin is a hormone produced in the pancreas, which aids in pushing the glucose from out blood to the necessary cells, reducing the blood sugar level and keeping it normal.**

A person who suffers from diabetes has high blood glucose levels. This is either caused by a lack of insulin production by the pancreas or the cells not responding to the insulin. This causes glucose level in the blood to rise. The excess glucose is eventually excreted from the body through urination, but your body reaps no benefits from it. This causes a metabolic slowdown.

The increased blood sugar level has a very large impact on your life.

Recurrent urination (polyuria), amplified thirst (polydipsia) and elevated hunger (polyphagia) are some of the most common effects felt by people who suffer from high blood glucose level.

If proper steps are not taken to prevent and control diabetes, the disease can have a very large impact on your life. The disease can have long term as well as short-term effects on your body.

Long-term effects could be conditions like damage to the eyes, kidney failure, foot ulcers, heart diseases, etc. Some of the more severe complications include nonketotic hyperosmolar coma and diabetic ketoacidosis.

Effect Of Diabetes On The Body

Diabetics have to take a lot of care of their body. High blood glucose levels slowly affect the nerves and lead to poor circulation. This results in slow healing of wounds, and if the wounds are not treated properly, they may get bacterial or fungal infections or even get gangrene and might eventually result in amputation.

The slow healing particularly affects the feet of diabetics and they are advised to check their feet on a regular basis and report any slow healing wound to a medical practitioner immediately.

Another effect of high glucose levels in the bloodstream is weight gain. And weight gain is a diabetic's worst enemy! Increased weight leads to spiked blood sugar levels, which can have a very negative impact on their overall health.

Chapter 2: What Are The Different Types Of Diabetes?

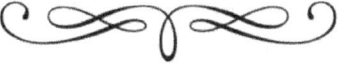

Diabetes can be broadly classified into three types based on the cause of the disease.

Type 1 Diabetes

Like we earlier mentioned, insulin is essential for the glucose to be absorbed by the cells for energy and growth.

Type 1 Diabetes occurs when the pancreas stops the production of insulin. This type of diabetes is also referred to as early-onset diabetes, insulin-dependent diabetes and juvenile diabetes.

The usual patients of Type 1 Diabetes get the disease before hitting their 40th birthday, often in their teens and early 20s.

Type 1 Diabetes is very uncommon, accounting for just 10% of the total diabetes cases worldwide!

Type 1 Diabetes patients need to take insulin injections for life, properly maintain their blood sugar levels, do regular blood tests and follow a special diet to ensure that they do not suffer harsh consequences.

According to a study conducted by the Centers for Disease Control and Prevention (CDC) the instances of type 1 diabetes occurrence in the youth under 20s has risen by about 23% in the United States.

Type 2 Diabetes

Type 2 Diabetes occurs gradually. At first, the body develops insulin resistance, a condition where the cells stop responding to the insulin and stop absorbing the glucose from the blood. Gradually, as the disease progresses, the body may even suffer from a lack of insulin.

This type of diabetes was earlier referred to as adult-onset diabetes and non insulin-dependent diabetes mellitus (NIDDM).

Type 2 Diabetes is the most common type of diabetes, accounting for almost 90% of the diabetes cases worldwide!

With a healthy diet and lifestyle, losing extra weight and regular monitoring of the blood sugar levels, an individual can control their diabetes. But, as Type 2 Diabetes is an extremely progressive disease that worsens over time, the patient might be required to take insulin tablets over a period of time.

People who are overweight and obese are at a higher risk of contracting Type 2 Diabetes, as compared to those who have the ideal body weight. At the highest risk are those people who have a large quantity of visceral fat, commonly known as abdominal fat, belly fat or central obesity.

But, why does fat have such a large impact on a person's chances of contracting Type 2 Diabetes? When you are overweight, the body releases certain chemicals, which weaken the body's metabolism and cardiovascular functions.

Another thing that affects the chances of contracting Type 2 Diabetes is an unhealthy diet. **According to a study conducted by the Imperial College London, the chances of developing type 2 diabetes increases by 22% due to the consumption of just one can of non diet soda per day!** This is how little unhealthy habits impact our overall health.

Another factor that influences the chances of getting Type 2 Diabetes is age. As we get older, our activity decreases. This lack of activity results in weight gain, which further results in an increased risk of type 2 diabetes.

According to the researchers at Edinburgh University, lower testosterone levels in a man can be linked to insulin resistance, which further leads to Type 2 Diabetes.

Gestational Diabetes

When pregnant, women need to take a lot of care. They are prone to a lot of diseases in their delicate condition, and it doesn't take a lot of time for the situation to complicate.

One such disease is gestational diabetes. **A very common condition during pregnancy, gestational diabetes occurs in about 2 to 10 percent of pregnant women.**

As we all know, when a woman gets pregnant, she goes through a lot of major hormonal changes. Sometimes, some of these hormonal changes result in insulin resistance and the cells stop responding to the insulin.

For most budding mothers, this isn't a problem. When the body requires extra insulin, the pancreas discharges more of it. But, when the pancreas cannot meet the insulin demands of the body, the blood sugar level rises, resulting in gestational diabetes.

Usually, after the baby is born, most women recover from gestational diabetes. In very few cases women continue being diabetic post pregnancy. Though, if a woman has suffered from gestational diabetes in her pregnancy, she is at an increased risk of suffering from gestational diabetes again in future pregnancies. The risk of suffering from regular diabetes also increases in the future.

Gestational diabetes can be controlled with a healthy diet and proper exercise routine. Only about 10 percent of women require blood sugar controlling medication.

Though pretty harmless, if the disease goes undiagnosed or gets out of control, it can cause complications during labor and the child may be bigger than normal.

According to the scientists from the National Institutes of Health and Harvard University, **women who consume a cholesterol rich and animal fat rich diet before getting pregnant are at a much higher risk of getting gestational diabetes**, as opposed to women who consume a low cholesterol and low animal fat diet before they got pregnant.

Chapter 3: Effects Of Different Types Of Food On A Diabetic's Body

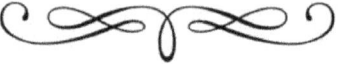

Food!! You can't live without it. Most of the times, diabetics are faced with the dilemma, of what to eat and what to avoid.

It is essential you understand how different foods and the quantities you consume affects glucose levels in your blood. **All foods contain varying levels of carbohydrates, proteins and fats, and all those nutrients have a very large impact on your blood glucose levels after you consume them**.

Carbohydrates

Carbohydrate or "carb" rich foods have the highest impact on your blood glucose levels. Carbs are present in all the starchy foods like pasta, potatoes, corn, bread, rice, cereals, etc., and in "sweet" foods like milk, sweets and yogurt. A lot of diets will suggest that you completely give up on carbs. This really isn't the way to go.

A lot of healthy foods contain starch and they really need to be included in your daily diet to ensure a healthy balanced diet.

Due to the large impact on your blood sugar levels, **starchy foods should not occupy more than one fourth of your meal**. Put in some rice on your plate, or a side of mashed potatoes, or a puree of corn, or even some lightly sauced pasta.

Protein

Protein is one of the building blocks of your body and performs many important functions, like providing your body with energy. Proteins have a very low impact on the blood sugar levels. Protein is usually found in most animal products, dairy products, beans and nuts.

As proteins have a very less effect on the blood glucose, it is advisable that at least one fourth of your meal consists of a protein rich food.

Add in a sausage or a piece of poached fish or even some lightly sautéed tofu.

Fats

Fat rich food **slow down the digestion process**, resulting in low blood sugar levels right after the meal, but increased blood glucose levels some time after the meal has been consumed.

Consuming healthier fats and restraining your high fat content foods can help reduce the risk of getting heart diseases. This is absolutely essential for people suffering from Type 2 Diabetes, as heart diseases are a major risk for them. Consumption of healthy fats should be done in moderation to ensure a reduced risk of heart diseases.

The other half of your meal should contain a variety of nutrient rich non-starchy vegetables like cauliflower, broccoli, carrots, tomatoes, string beans, etc. Add in a refreshing citrus rich salad, to add some texture as well as some uplifting flavors to your meal.

These won't increase or decrease your blood sugar levels, but will provide you with a balanced meal, something that will ensure that you don't gain weight and aggravate your blood sugar levels even more.

It is very important that you consume balanced meals and make sure your blood sugar levels remain in control.

Chapter 4: Diabetes 101: Which Foods And Drinks Diabetics Should Consume And Avoid?

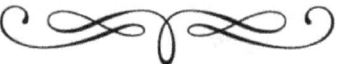

If you have diabetes it doesn't mean you need to starve or stay away from all your favorite foods or even consume tasteless and boring food for life. This said you can't eat everything in sight. With a little restraint and you will be able to consume a lot of the foods you thought were out of bounds.

Foods And Drinks To Avoid

The foods and drinks that we have listed in our "**Foods and Drinks To Avoid**" list have a high content of sodium, calories, carbohydrates, saturated fats and may even contain the dreaded trans fats!

Foods with high sugar, carbohydrate and calories content can lead to unsolicited weight gain and spikes in blood glucose levels. Foods with high sodium and saturated fat content can increase the dangers of contracting heart diseases.

All of this is can really increase the risks of complications while suffering from diabetes.

Yes, this list may contain some of the foods that you really relish and love to gorge down. Don't worry, we have provided you with healthier substitutes, which will ensure you don't need to give up your favorite tastes altogether.

For example: If you love consuming French fries, you can still continue eating them, but with a minor alteration. Instead of eating the deep fried version, opt for the healthier baked one and you will be good to go!

Nachos

Often, we walk into restaurants and order a side of nachos with our meal to satiate our hunger until our food arrives. **Did you know that nachos often contain and sometimes even exceed the calorific, carbohydrate and fat content of an entire meal!**

Opt for baked nachos instead of fried ones and ditch your regular cheese sauce for a healthier low fat cheese sauce. Top your nachos with some avocados. Treat a plate of nachos as a complete meal as opposed to the side appetizer it is usually considered to be.

Coffee and Its Variants

Most coffee-shop beverages can knock a lot full fledges desserts out of the park with their high sugar, carb, fat and calorific content. And as a diabetic, this can spell really bad news for you!

A plain old coffee, with very little milk or a half and half combination, is a healthier choice for you. Or you could opt for a cup of green tea! It is healthier and prevents heart diseases and even cancer to some extent!

Biscuits and Sausage Gravy

According to the American Diabetes Association, it is advisable to consume less than 7 percent of your daily calories from saturated fats. For an average person, this is about 15 grams per day.

But, did you know, the average biscuits and sausage gravy meal contains 13 grams of saturated fats. Your day's fat content in a single meal!

Substitute the ingredients in the traditional breakfast dish. Use cheddar biscuits instead of the regular biscuits, or even crisp some chicken in the oven and use it instead! You will have a delicious meal on your hands without the added saturated fats and sodium.

Fried Fish

Usually, fish is one of the healthiest foods for any diabetic. After all, they have a very low fat content and are rich in nutrients.

But, this depends a lot on how the fish is prepared. Baked fish with a salad? Good. Steamed fish dumplings? Really good. Deep fried breaded fish with a side of fries and hushpuppies and coleslaw? Not good at all!

A typical fish platter contains two large filets of deep fried fish, some deep fried French fries and hushpuppies, and a side of coleslaw. Typically, it contains about 3000 milligrams of sodium, double the quantity of the prescribed daily sodium limit for a diabetic!

Instead, opt for a plate of baked or grilled fish, which makes up for about one fourths of your plate's content, some starchy vegetables like baked or boiled potatoes occupying the other one fourth. For the remaining half of your plate, fill it up with some non-starchy veggies and you'll have a delicious, healthy meal to gorge down!

Pre-Packaged Fruit Juices Or Fruit Beverages

Fruits are healthy and natural, so shouldn't they be good for your health? Yes and no. Most pre-packaged juices contain sweeteners that add extra sugar to your diet.

Make it a point to read the labels and gauge for yourself the amount of sugar you want to be consuming.

Keep in mind, most pre-packaged beverage labels show the nutritional content for a single serving to fool you into thinking that the whole bottle has a limited sugar content.

Don't be fooled. The single serve size is almost one fourth of the total content of the bottle or tetra pack!

Leave behind the unnaturally flavored beverages and rather go for fresh fruit juices you can make in your juicer at home. **Make it a point to not add any extra sugar or sweetener to your juice.**

You could even muddle some fruit in a pitcher, top with some chilled water and leave in the fridge for a while. **Fruit infused water has a delicate sweet flavor to it and doesn't feel too overpowering, in terms of flavor and texture, either.**

Frozen Meals

Life has become so busy, who has the time to cook? Pre-packaged, frozen meals are your best bet for providing yourself and your family "home cooked" meals.

These frozen meals are full of preservatives and unhealthy levels of fats and sodium, which can be unhealthy for both, you and your family!

Always check the label and pick a meal with less than 400 grams of calories. Also make sure the sodium content is not more than 600 milligrams and the saturated fat doesn't exceed 4 grams.

Another handy tip is keep chopped up veggies in your freezer. Every time you cook a frozen meal, add some of the frozen veggies to it before you start cooking. They not only will increase the nutritional value of your meal, they will also increase the portion size, without adding extra calories to your meal.

Soda or Fizzy Drinks

According to a study conducted by the Imperial College of London, **a 12-ounce serving of sugar-sweetened beverages can up the risk of getting diabetes by 20%.** Imagine the devastation it can cause to your already spiked up blood sugar levels!

Instead, settle for a glass of regular water. If you really need a quick sugar fix, have some fruit infused water or natural, non-sweetened fruit juice instead!

Foods and Drinks to Consume

Food is the one thing that you a diabetic need to exercise extreme control over; after all, one wrong food and you could be stuck with a spiked up blood sugar and an increased heart disease risk!

Along with the foods you should avoid, it is essential to know the foods you should consume. As discussed in an earlier chapter, proteins do not have much of an effect on blood sugar levels, so it is advisable to incorporate a lot of proteins in your diet.

You do not need to necessarily consume exotic, hard to find stuff. Pick foods that are high in fiber and minerals and you could be consuming healthy meals in no time!

Our list of "Foods and Drinks to Consume" contains a list of healthy, high fiber and antioxidant rich foods, which will satiate you as well as keep your body healthy.

Apples

"An apple a day keeps the doctor away," and rightly said so! According to a study published in Journal of Functional Foods by the Ohio State University, eating an apple every day, for four weeks in a row, reduces the bad cholesterol in your body.

So, trade in your evening snack of chips for a delicious apple. When you make dessert, add apples as a sweetener, instead of sugar. Apples can be used in a wide variety of dishes, making them healthy and delicious!

Asparagus

According to Charles Lamb "**Asparagus inspires gentle thoughts,**" and why wouldn't it? In a research published in the British Nutrition Journal, researchers claim that asparagus controls blood glucose levels and increases insulin levels in our body.

This makes it every diabetic's best friend!

Low on calories, asparagus contains only 20 calories per 5 grams and contains and even provides our body with 33 percent of the recommended folate content.

Now wonder it inspires gentle thoughts, considering it balances so many inconsistencies in our body!

Dark Chocolate

9 out of 10 people like chocolate and the 10th person always lies. Well maybe not. But, our point here is, a lot of people love chocolate.

Along with being absolutely delicious, chocolate is a rich source of flavonoids. **Dark chocolate also contains a lot of nutrients that reduces the insulin resistance of your body and improves cell insulin sensitivity.** It even mutes a lot of your unhealthy cravings!

If all this wasn't enough, chocolate even reduces the risk of heart diseases by calming your blood pressure, further reducing the risk of strokes. But, this doesn't mean you eat any chocolate you can get your hands on.

Limited consumption of dark chocolate over a period of 5 years reduces the risk of getting a heart attack by 2 percent.

Fish

As opposed to other meats, sea food has a less content of saturated fats and cholesterol. **Fatty fishes, like halibut, salmon, sardines, etc., are a great source of omega 3 fatty acids.** The omega 3 fatty acids help reduce blood pressure and control inflammation.

Grill it, steam it, bake it or lightly fry it – fish can be incorporated in your diet in various forms. The serving size for fish is the same as other meat and poultry, 3 ounces.

Yes, ordering fish can be a bit more expensive, but buying raw fish and making it at home can be a far cheaper option! Make a salad or a sandwich or grill the whole fish with a seasoning, your possibilities are endless!

Melon

There various amounts of melons available in the produce section of your local market. The next time you crave something sweet head there and grab one of these nutrient rich, delicious fruits.

Watermelon

Watermelon is a great **source of antioxidants**, which may help prevent a lot of cancers and reduces the cell damage which is usually associated with heart diseases. Watermelon has a very low saturated fat content and is quite satiating. Trade in your mid-morning snack for a healthy bowl of cubed watermelon.

Honeydew

Very rich in Vitamin C, a 1 cup serving of honeydew melons fulfills about 51% of your daily vitamin C content quite effortlessly.

Like watermelon, the honeydew melon has a great satiating capacity. The honeydew melon fills your tummy without adding a lot of calories to your diet.

Cantaloupe

This mouthwatering melon provides you with double nutrition. Rich in Vitamin A and Vitamin C, it improves vision and reduces macular degeneration.

Nuts

Most nuts are rich in omega 3 fatty acids, vitamin E and unsaturated fats that make your artery walls flexible and reduce the chances of getting blood clots.

Nuts also help in controlling blood glucose and bad cholesterol levels.

It is extremely easy to incorporate nuts in your meals. Chop up some walnuts, roast them and add them to your salad for an extra crunch. **Substitute the milk in your dishes with some almond milk for some added taste**. Nuts add an added flavor as well as nutritional boost to your meals.

Spinach

As a child you often saw Popeye guzzling spinach before beating Bluto black and blue and dreamed of doing so too!

Well, Popeye did get something right! Spinach is laden with a variety of vitamins and minerals.

The non-starchy green veggie has a very low carbohydrate and calorific value, while having a really high vitamin C and folate value.

Need another reason to consume spinach? **According to a report by the American Diabetes Association, regularly eating green leafy veggies reduces the chances of an individual contracting Type 2 Diabetes by 14 percent.**

Using spinach in your meals is just not limited to salads. Finely chop some spinach and add it to your scrambled egg. Or layer it to make lasagna. Add some lightly fried spinach to your plate as a side with some crispy chicken. The possibilities are endless!

Tea

Despite the popular notion that green tea is healthier than regular black tea, a research by the Antioxidants Research Laboratory at the Jean Mayer USDA Human Nutrition Research Center on Aging at Tufts University has shown that the nutritional and health benefits are pretty similar each other.

The study even goes on to suggest that drinking four to five cups of strong tea daily can be quite beneficial. But be warned, this doesn't apply to bottled teas. The beneficial catechins start degrading once the tea is prepared, and the bottled tea may contain a lot of preservatives and extra sugar in it.

Tea only contains half the amount of caffeine found in coffee, and is a much healthier option than any other beverages that just add empty calories to your body.

Chapter 5: Suggested Healthy Activities And Exercises

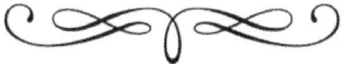

It is very important for people with diabetes to exercise. Regularly exercising not only helps keep blood glucose levels in control, but also helps reduce the risk of heart diseases.

But why is it so? The explanation is quite simple. Like we explained earlier, glucose is one of the energy providers for your body.

When you move around, exercise and do physical activities, your muscles use up more glucose, hence reducing the glucose in your bloodstream.

Exercising has an added benefit of weight loss, a thing that is absolutely essential for people with diabetes. Physical activity also reduces the stress build up in your body and provides a healthy outlet for all your pent up stress.

What is exercise?

Exercise is any moderately intense activity that is **performed for at least 150 minutes per week**. Aerobic activity with restrained power means exercising to the degree that your heart rate rises to a certain extent and makes your start perspiring.

This can include a variety of activities, which can pertain to but are not limited to:

- Brisk walking
- Slow jogging
- Riding a bike
- Rowing with manual oars
- Sports like: table tennis, lawn tennis, badminton, racquetball, squash, etc.
- Swimming exercises: water aerobics, water polo, swimming, etc.

You don't need to specifically do sports or such activities in an effort to exercise. Some of your day-to-day activities, with a little alteration, can be counted as exercise.

Instead of using a motorized lawn mower use a manual one to mow your lawn. When you go shopping, carry your bags around instead of using a trolley to push your stuff around.

When you take your dog out for a walk, brisk walk instead of leisurely walking; increase the time duration of your walks so that it can count towards your exercise.

You need to try and reduce your "sedentary" activities. Sitting or lying down for long durations can be very bad for your health. Such activities just increase your weight, which in turn can up your chances of getting chronic heart diseases.

Chapter 6: 30-Day Suggested Meal Plan

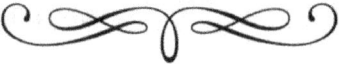

Breakfast

"Never work before breakfast. If you have to work before breakfast, get your breakfast first." - Josh Billings

We have often heard that breakfast is one of the most important meals of the day. A healthy refreshing start to the day is ideal for an energized day. **If you skip breakfast, you spend the entire day feeling down. But if you start your day with a refreshing meal, it will keep up your pace and energy all day long.**

But, starting your day with something unhealthy is unadvisable. Fill your meal with lots of fresh fruits and vegetables to ensure you are not weighed down by a lot of carbohydrates first thing in the day.

Lunch

Your lunch marks your mid-day meal. You should make sure that is healthy and invigorating. A very heavy and carb rich lunch can make you feel sleepy and lethargic.

Make sure your lunch contains a balanced proportion of proteins, carbohydrates, fats and fibers.

Do not skip your lunch, especially if you're working. Skipping meals has a very negative impact on your body and causes problems like acidity. And you may end up gorging on unhealthy processed foods to compensate for the lost meal.

Dinner

"Breakfast like a king, lunch like a prince and dinner like a pauper," they say. As your day progresses, it is advisable that you reduce your carb intake.

This in no way means that you skip your dinner or just make do with a glass of milk for the night. **Your meal needs to be satiating enough to last you through the night, but not too heavy on your stomach.**

It is advisable you **eat your meal at least 3 hours before you sleep**, so that your food digests well. Your digestion process slows down for the night and it is preferable that your food gets digested before you fall asleep.

Here is a suggested 30-Day Plan:

Day 1

Breakfast: Whole grain bagel with some lightly sautéed fresh fruit and a cup of fat free milk.

Lunch: Bacon, lettuce and tomato salad with whole wheat pita bread and an orange.

Dinner: Roasted salmon with a side of Afrikano spiced carrots and cinnamon spiced apple.

Day2

Breakfast: Fat free yogurt with granola cereal, flaxseed and chopped nuts.

Lunch: Shiitake mushroom and basil fettuccini and skimmed milk.

Dinner: Cajun chicken croquets, steamed asparagus and fennel salad.

Day 3

Breakfast: Whole grain English muffin, with scrambled egg with tomato and onion, and a cup of fat free milk.

Lunch: Pan roasted corn, black bean and mango salad, turkey quesadillas and an apple.

Dinner: Boiled lentils with grilled sandwich, julienne vegetable stir fry and melon.

Day4

Breakfast: Fate free yogurt with chopped fresh fruits and nuts.

Lunch: Chicken and orange salad with whole wheat bread toast and fresh fruit smoothie.

Dinner: Slow cooked lamb and vegetable stew with brown rice and plain yogurt.

Day 5

Breakfast: Oatmeal with roasted and chopped walnuts and a cup of calcium enriched soy milk or fat free milk.

Lunch: Roasted chicken wings, apricot and skimmed milk.

Dinner: Pan cooked pork with a low sugar cranberry sauce, baby carrots and nutty green leafy vegetable salad.

Day 6

Breakfast: Bagel and low fat cream cheese with a cup of rice beverage or fat free milk.

Lunch: Chicken and bulgur tabbouleh with a sliced tomato and pepper salad and low fat milk.

Dinner: Irish style lamb stew with a Hawaiian smoothie.

Day 7

Breakfast: Spinach, mushroom and onion omelet with a whole wheat bread toast and a cup of green tea.

Lunch: Tropical fruit and tuna salad with a whole wheat pita bread.

Dinner: Grilled broccoli with lemon, whole wheat couscous and one cup cantaloupe.

Day 8

Breakfast: Cheerios cereal with fat free milk and a medium orange.

Lunch: Roasted vegetable pasta, winter greens salad and an apricot.

Dinner: Grilled salmon with African Piri Piri sauce, brown rice and steamed broccoli.

Day 9

Breakfast: Bran flake cereal, fresh banana and skimmed milk.

Lunch: Tomato and Turkey Panini and fresh fruit juice.

Dinner: Roasted pork loin with a rosemary and plum jus and a whole wheat couscous.

Day 10

Breakfast: Whole wheat English muffin with low fat cream cheese, blueberries and low fat milk.

Lunch: Greek style lemon rice soup, whole wheat pita bread and skimmed milk.

Dinner: Grilled coffee flavored steak, wild rice, steamed broccoli and fresh mango sorbet.

Day 11

Breakfast: Corn tortilla with scrambled egg, a plum and skimmed milk.

Lunch: Salmon burger, with zucchini soup and low fat milk.

Dinner: Shallow fried turkey cutlet with glazed carrots and buttermilk mashed potatoes.

Day 12

Breakfast: Whole grain flake cereal, skimmed milk and a kiwi.

Lunch: Chicken and rice soup, spinach and raspberry salad, whole wheat bread and watermelon.

Dinner: Curry flavored shrimp with orange segments, brown rice and raspberries.

Day 13

Breakfast: Oatmeal bran bread with scrambled egg, grapefruit and 1% milk.

Lunch: Tomato and red onion soup with yogurt and cilantro, whole wheat bread and honeydew melon.

Dinner: Grilled chicken with barbeque sauce.

Day 14

Breakfast: Whole wheat English muffin with creamy peanut butter and sugar free jam and low fat milk.

Lunch: Spiced pork stuffed in lettuce wraps, whole wheat bread and papaya salad.

Dinner: Sliced roast beef with brown rice and a pear.

Day15

Breakfast: Oatmeal with apple slices and cinnamon.

Lunch: Egg soup with sautéed asparagus and avocado and mango salad.

Dinner: Baked halibut with roasted onion and peppers.

Day 16

Breakfast: Whole wheat English muffin with strawberries, almond butter and unsweetened coconut flakes.

Lunch: Lentil soup, green leafy vegetable salad and whole bran toast.

Dinner: Whole grain pasta with turkey meat balls and an apricot.

Day 17

Breakfast: Fat free vanilla yogurt and blueberry and strawberry parfait topped with grated toasted coconut.

Lunch: Sautéed thyme fish filets with green salad and whole wheat toast.

Dinner: Brown rice and shrimps with whole wheat bread toast.

Day 18

Breakfast: Egg and Ham stuffed corn tortillas with fat free cheddar cheese.

Lunch: Roasted pepper, tuna and whole wheat pasta salad, whole wheat pita bread and low fat milk.

Dinner: Grilled chicken with three bean salad.

Day 19

Breakfast: Tomato and Spinach Baked Egg with skimmed milk.

Lunch: Gnocchi with zucchini and parsley butter and an orange.

Dinner: Tofu and vegetable stir-fry, whole wheat pita bread and watermelon.

Day 20

Breakfast: Whole wheat toast, with sugar free plum spread and a fresh fruit smoothie.

Lunch: Whole wheat vegetable burger and an apricot.

Dinner: Poached salmon fillets, arugula salad and strawberries.

Day 21

Breakfast: Tofu stuffed scrambled egg with whole wheat toast and strawberries.

Lunch: Rice and Pinto bean salad with whole wheat pita bread and dark chocolate and pistachio butter sandwich.

Dinner: Grilled pork tenderloin with brown rice and lettuce salad with creamy orange dressing.

Day 22

Breakfast: Muesli with fresh cranberries and low fat milk.

Lunch: Brown rice with ham and egg frittata and fresh pineapple.

Dinner: Barbeque flavored pork loin, brown rice and spinach salad with an olive vinaigrette.

Day 23

Breakfast: Whole wheat toast with roasted apple butter and fresh apricot smoothie.

Lunch: Chicken and Greek yogurt salad with vegetables, and whole wheat bread.

Dinner: Pesto rubbed lamb, whole wheat couscous, steamed broccoli and apricot.

Day 24

Breakfast: Asparagus and cheese frittata with an apple and skimmed milk.

Lunch: Salmon and lentil salad with whole wheat pita bread.

Dinner: Grilled steak and peppers, oven baked sweet potato fries and peach and lime sorbet.

Day 25

Breakfast: Blueberry almond flour pancakes with low fat ricotta spread, a fresh banana and low fat milk.

Lunch: Tuna and green olive salad with whole grain wheat crackers.

Dinner: Garlic flavored pork loin with a shredded coconut and carrot salad and raspberries.

Day 26

Breakfast: Vegetable quiche, whole wheat bread toast and skimmed milk.

Lunch: Crisp tortilla with baked pinto bean and low fat Mexican blend cheese spread.

Dinner: Ginger and coconut flavored roasted chicken with steamed cauliflower and frozen strawberry yogurt.

Day 27

Breakfast: Apricot oatmeal and low fat milk.

Lunch: Whole grain roasted beef sandwich with tomatoes.

Dinner: Chili flavored steak with brown rice and steamed spinach and peach.

Day 28

Breakfast: Plain yogurt, whole wheat bread toast and roasted pear butter.

Lunch: Chicken, grape and green leafy vegetable salad and whole wheat bread toast.

Dinner: Shrimp with a whole wheat roll, whole wheat pita bread and lettuce and cucumber salad.

Day29

Breakfast: Baked vegetable ragout with egg and skimmed milk.

Lunch: Garbanzo bean and green leafy veggie salad and a fresh peach.

Dinner: Vegetable and chicken stew with whole wheat bread, a tangerine and skimmed milk.

Day 30

Breakfast: Blueberry and corn muffins with fresh strawberries and low fat milk.

Lunch: Whole wheat English muffin topped with tuna and low fat mayonnaise and a cup fat free milk and a side of baby carrots.

Dinner: Pan fried chicken in a sweet apricot sauce, brown rice, parboiled asparagus and a mango.

Conclusion

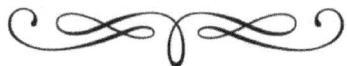

I hope this book was able to help you to find meaningful and effective ways to bring your diabetes under control.

The next step is to make sure that you follow the tips provided in this book. Remember, if you are suffering from diabetes, it is very important that make sure you eat healthy, exercise well and most of all take care of yourself.

Do not over indulge and exercise some control on your portion sizes. Just because you are allowed to eat a certain type of food, it doesn't mean you gorge down boxes of that particular food.

Once again we would like to remind you to not embark on any diet plan before consulting your physician and discussing your meal plan with them in great detail.

I hope the content of this book was helpful to you and you enjoyed reading it.

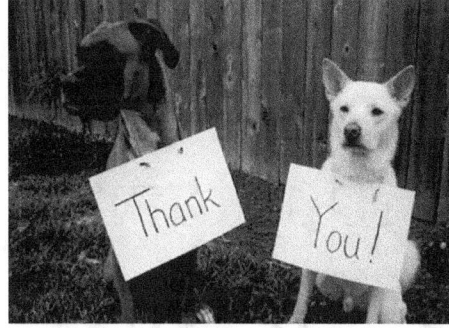

Finally, if you enjoyed this book, then I'd like to ask you for a favor, would you be kind enough to leave a review for this book on Amazon? It'd be greatly appreciated!

Thank you and good luck!

Jamie Tyler

If you're interested in learning more about Gluten-free Diet and Lifestyle and free preview of upcoming books? Please sign up for my Gluten-free Lifestyle Newsletter and receive these gifts FREE!

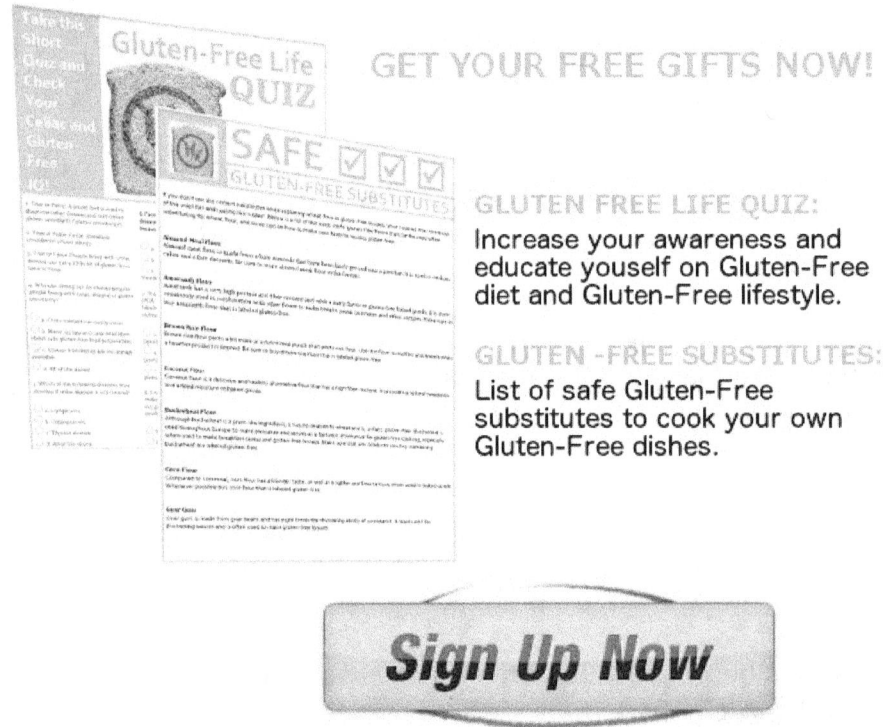

GET YOUR FREE GIFTS NOW!

GLUTEN FREE LIFE QUIZ:

Increase your awareness and educate youself on Gluten-Free diet and Gluten-Free lifestyle.

GLUTEN -FREE SUBSTITUTES:

List of safe Gluten-Free substitutes to cook your own Gluten-Free dishes.

VISIT THIS LINK TO GET YOUR GIFTS:

http://bit.ly/1zVbPGw

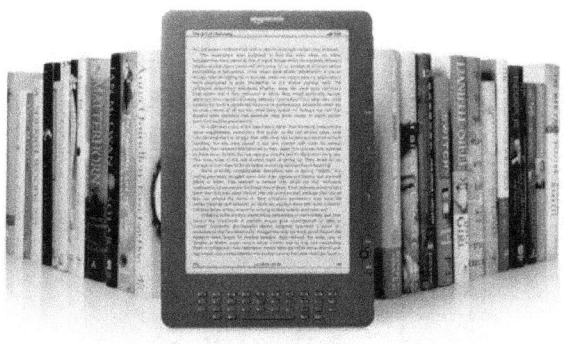

Gluten Free Snacks: 50 Incredible Gluten-Free Snack Recipes for Gluten-Free Family

Gluten Free Vegan: Healthy Vegetarian Gluten Free Recipes: Vegan, Animal Free Breakfast, Lunch and Dinner Recipes

Gluten Free: Beginner Guide to Everything Gluten-Free: Gluten-Free Diet and Gluten-Free Recipes: Easy Recipes, Suggestions and Guide to Eating Healthy and Cheap

Diabetic Diet: 30-Day Lifestyle Plan To Maintain A Healthy Weight: Weight Loss And Healthy Diet Plan For Diabetics

Lose Weight: 30-Day Lifestyle Plan to Better Health by Losing Weight: What To and Not To Eat, Drink, & Making Lifestyle Changes To Look Amazing And Feel Great

Divorce With Children: Recovering From Divorce And Putting Your Life Back On Track: Dealing With Divorce, Your Ex, Children And Everything In Between

Parenting For Single Mothers: Being A Good Mom And Raising Great Kids

Raising Girls with ADHD: 20 Lessons and Tips for Parents: Tips and Strategies For Parents Dealing With Raising A Daughter With ADHD

Raising Boys With ADHD: 20 Lessons and Tips for Parents

DIY: Top 50 Hacks for Home Cleaning

Gluten Free Desserts: 50 Incredible Gluten-Free Snack Recipes for Gluten-Free Family

Sugar Free Recipes: 25 Delicious Breakfast, Lunch, and Dinner Easy Sugar-Free Recipes (Sugar Detox Diet)

Weight Watchers: Simple Quick Start Easy Recipes for Breakfast, Lunch, and Dinner

FREE Kindle Books and New Kindle Book Announcements!

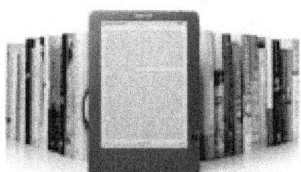

Join our exclusive readers club and receive notification when our books are FREE on Kindle Store for limited time. Also be the first to know about exciting new titles that are published every month for only $0.99.

*** We hate spam and never share your email with anyone ***

JOIN NOW!

VISIT THIS LINK TO JOIN:
http://bit.ly/1AtBHOU